CIALIS (TADALAFIL) USAGE GUIDE FOR MEN

A Practical Guide To Taking Cialis Safely

Dr. Hilda Tomlin

DISCLAIMER

Disclaimer

This Cialis Usage Guide For Men is for informational purposes only and does not replace professional medical advice, diagnosis, or treatment. Always consult your healthcare provider with questions regarding your health or medications. Individual responses to Levitra may vary, and this guide does not guarantee results. The authors and publishers are not responsible for any adverse effects resulting from the use of the information contained in this guide.

Table of Contents

Introduction

In this chapter, we will explore Cialis, a medication for managing erectile dysfunction (ED) and certain urinary symptoms associated with benign prostatic hyperplasia (BPH). Known for its active ingredient, tadalafil, Cialis is part of a class of drugs called PDE5 inhibitors, which enhance blood flow to specific areas of the body. Unlike some alternatives, Cialis offers a longer duration of action, earning it the nickname "the weekend pill."

This chapter highlights its unique features, including its extended effectiveness, and its dual approval for ED and BPH. understanding its mechanism and limitations is essential for safe and effective use.

In this guide, we aim to provide an informative and practical resource for anyone considering or currently using Cialis. From understanding how it works to recognizing potential side effects and interactions, this guide offers a comprehensive overview tailored to your needs.

We focus on providing balanced, factual information to help you make informed decisions about your health. It is essential to use it as part of a broader strategy, which may include lifestyle changes and medical advice, for optimal results. This guide is not a substitute for professional medical consultation but rather a complement to it.

What is Cialis?

In this chapter, we will focus on Cialis, a prescription medication primarily used to treat erectile dysfunction (ED) and the urinary symptoms of benign prostatic hyperplasia (BPH). Its active ingredient, tadalafil, is a PDE5 inhibitor that works by relaxing blood vessels and improving blood flow to specific areas of the body, such as the penis. This mechanism helps men achieve and maintain erections when sexually stimulated and alleviates BPH-related discomfort.

It is also approved for daily use in lower doses for individuals who prefer ongoing management of their condition. Iis essential to approach its use responsibly and with a thorough understanding of its benefits and limitations.

It is important to note that Cialis does not cure ED or BPH but helps manage the symptoms when used as prescribed. Its effectiveness and safety depend on individual health factors and proper usage, which will be explored in detail in later chapters.

Before starting Cialis, discuss with a professional medical pactictional.

Mechanism of Action

In this chapter, we will discuss the mechanism of action of Cialis, which is based on its active ingredient, tadalafil. Cialis is a phosphodiesterase type 5 (PDE5) inhibitor, a class of drugs designed to enhance blood flow in specific areas of the body.

The process begins with sexual stimulation, which triggers the release of nitric oxide (NO) in the blood vessels of the penis. Nitric oxide stimulates the production of cyclic guanosine monophosphate (cGMP), a chemical that relaxes smooth muscle cells and widens blood vessels, allowing increased blood flow. This enhanced blood flow is essential for achieving and maintaining an erection.

Tadalafil works by inhibiting the PDE5 enzyme, which is responsible for breaking down cGMP. By blocking this enzyme, Cialis ensures higher levels of cGMP remain in the system, sustaining the blood vessel relaxation needed for effective erections.

For individuals with benign prostatic hyperplasia (BPH), tadalafil relaxes the muscles in the prostate and bladder, alleviating symptoms like frequent or difficult urination.

Cialis requires sexual stimulation to initiate this biochemical process, and its effects can last up to 36 hours, offering extended flexibility. However, the duration and effectiveness depend on individual factors, including overall health and concurrent medications. Always seek medical advice to understand how this mechanism applies to your situation.

Indications and Uses of Cialis

In this chapter, we will discuss the primary medical purposes of Cialis, focusing on its approved uses in managing specific health conditions.

1. Erectile Dysfunction (ED)

Cialis is used in managing erectile dysfunction, a condition that can impact a person's ability to achieve or maintain an erection during sexual activity. By enhancing blood flow to the penile tissue, it may help improve erectile function when combined with sexual stimulation.

2. Benign Prostatic Hyperplasia (BPH)

It may be used to manage benign prostatic hyperplasia, a condition involving the enlargement of the prostate gland. Symptoms such as frequent urination, difficulty starting urination, or weak urine flow can sometimes be alleviated through the medication's action of relaxing smooth muscles in the prostate and bladder.

3. **Dual Use for ED and BPH**

For individuals experiencing both erectile dysfunction and symptoms of benign prostatic hyperplasia, Cialis may provide relief by addressing both conditions simultaneously.

Decisions regarding its use should always be made in consultation with a qualified healthcare provider.

Available Dosages

In this chapter, we discuss the different dosages and forms of Cialis, providing an overview of its commonly prescribed options. These variations allow for tailored treatment based on individual medical needs and conditions.

Available Dosages

Cialis is available in several dosages to accommodate various therapeutic needs:

- **2.5 mg**: Typically prescribed for daily use to maintain consistent levels of the medication in the body.

- **5 mg**: Often used for daily therapy, particularly for men who require ongoing management of erectile dysfunction (ED) or benign prostatic hyperplasia (BPH).

- **10 mg**: A standard dose for as-needed use, typically taken before anticipated sexual activity.

- **20 mg**: The highest dose, prescribed for as-needed use, and generally recommended for individuals who do not respond to lower doses.

It is essential to follow a healthcare provider's guidance regarding the appropriate dosage and form, as factors like age, underlying health conditions, and concurrent medications can influence the choice. Self-adjusting the dosage is not recommended, as it can lead to reduced effectiveness or an increased risk of side effects.

How to Use Cialis Safely

In this chapter, we explore guidelines for using Cialis effectively to manage conditions such as erectile dysfunction (ED) and benign prostatic hyperplasia (BPH). Proper use ensures the best possible outcomes while minimizing risks.

1. Timing and Dosage

- **For As-Needed Use**: Take Cialis at least 30 minutes before anticipated sexual activity. Its effects can last up to 36 hours, offering flexibility.

- **For Daily Use**: Take at the same time each day, regardless of sexual activity. This approach maintains a steady level of the medication in your body.

2. **Taking the Medication:** Swallow the tablet whole with water. heavy meals might delay its onset of action.

3. **Avoiding Overuse:** Do not take more than one dose per day. If using a daily dose, ensure consistency and avoid skipping doses without consulting your healthcare provider.

4. **Lifestyle Considerations:** Avoid excessive alcohol consumption, as it may reduce the effectiveness of Cialis and increase the risk of side effects. Grapefruit and grapefruit juice may interfere with how Cialis works, so these should be avoided unless otherwise advised by a doctor.

5. **Monitoring and Adjustments:** Keep track of how your body responds to Cialis and report any concerns to your healthcare provider. If the medication does not seem effective, do not adjust the dose on your own; consult a doctor for guidance.

Potential Side Effects

In this chapter, we address the potential side effects of Cialis, helping users recognize possible adverse reactions. While many individuals tolerate the medication well, side effects can occur and vary in intensity.

- **Headache**: This is one of the most frequently reported side effects and may be mild to moderate.

- **Flushing**: A warm sensation, often in the face, neck, or chest, can occur after taking Cialis.

- **Indigestion**: Some users experience upset stomach or acid reflux.

- **Nasal Congestion**: Stuffy or blocked nose is a common but temporary reaction.

- **Muscle Pain**: Mild discomfort, particularly in the back or limbs, is occasionally reported.

- **Dizziness**: Some users may feel lightheaded, particularly when standing up suddenly.

- **Vision Changes**: Rarely, individuals experience changes in color perception or blurred vision.

- **Hearing Changes**: Sudden hearing loss or ringing in the ears has been noted in rare cases.

- **Prolonged Erection (Priapism)**: An erection lasting more than four hours requires immediate medical attention to prevent permanent damage.

- **Chest Pain**: This could indicate a serious condition and should be evaluated by a healthcare professional.

- **Severe Allergic Reactions**: Swelling, difficulty breathing, or skin rashes require urgent care.

Always report any unusual or severe reactions to your healthcare provider.

How to Manage Side Effects

In this chapter, we discuss how to manage potential side effects when using Cialis. While side effects are generally mild and temporary, it is important to address them appropriately to ensure comfort and safety.

1. **Headache**: Over-the-counter may help relieve headaches. Staying hydrated and taking Cialis with food may reduce the likelihood of headaches.

2. **Flushing**: If flushing occurs, rest in a cool environment and drink water. It typically resolves on its own within a few hours. Avoid alcohol, which can exacerbate flushing, and take Cialis with a meal to reduce this effect.

3. **Indigestion** : Antacids may help ease indigestion symptoms. Avoid large, heavy meals before taking Cialis, and consider taking the medication with a light meal to minimize stomach discomfort.

4. **Nasal Congestion:** Nasal decongestants, such as saline sprays or antihistamines, may help clear the nasal passages. Taking Cialis at a lower dose may reduce the occurrence of this side effect.

5. **Muscle or Back Pain:** Gentle stretching, hydration, and over-the-counter pain relief can help alleviate muscle discomfort. Regular physical activity and maintaining good posture may minimize muscle pain while using Cialis.

6. **Dizziness**: If dizziness occurs, sit or lie down until the feeling passes. Avoid standing up quickly to prevent sudden drops in blood pressure. Staying hydrated and taking the medication as prescribed can reduce dizziness.

7. **Severe Side Effects**: For rare but serious side effects like priapism (prolonged erection), chest pain, or severe allergic reactions, immediate medical attention is required. Do not attempt to manage these side effects at home. Call emergency services if you experience any of these serious reactions.

If you experience side effects that persist or worsen, consult your healthcare provider for further advice on adjusting your dosage or exploring alternative treatments.

Drug Interactions

In this chapter, we explore the potential drug interactions that may occur when taking Cialis. Understanding these interactions is crucial to ensuring the safety and effectiveness of the medication.

1. **Nitrates:** Cialis should not be used with nitrate medications, which are commonly prescribed for chest pain (angina) or heart problems. The combination can lead to a dangerous drop in blood pressure, causing dizziness, fainting, or even a heart attack. Nitrates include medications like nitroglycerin, isosorbide dinitrate, and isosorbide mononitrate.

2. **Alpha-Blockers:** Alpha-blockers, used to treat high blood pressure and symptoms of BPH, can also lower

blood pressure. When taken with Cialis, they may increase the risk of low blood pressure, dizziness, or fainting. Examples include tamsulosin, alfuzosin, and doxazosin.

3. **Antifungals and Antibacterials:** Certain antifungals (e.g., ketoconazole) and antibiotics (e.g., erythromycin) can increase the concentration of Cialis in the blood, potentially leading to side effects such as headaches, back pain, or dizziness. It is important to adjust the Cialis dose when these drugs are prescribed together.

4. **HIV Protease Inhibitors:** HIV medications like ritonavir and lopinavir can increase Cialis levels, leading to an increased risk of side effects. A lower dose of Cialis may be recommended to reduce this risk.

5. **Other PDE5 Inhibitors:** Using Cialis with other PDE5 inhibitors (such as sildenafil or vardenafil) can increase the risk of side effects like headaches, dizziness, and priapism. These medications should not be taken together.

6. **Blood Pressure Medications:** When combined with other blood pressure medications, Cialis may amplify the blood pressure-lowering effects, leading to symptoms like lightheadedness, fainting, or dizziness. If you are taking blood pressure medication, it is crucial to monitor your blood pressure regularly.

7. **Grapefruit and Grapefruit Juice:** Grapefruit and grapefruit juice may interfere with the metabolism of Cialis, leading to higher levels of the drug in the bloodstream, which could increase the likelihood of side effects.

8. **Alcohol:** Excessive alcohol consumption can intensify some of the side effects of Cialis, such as dizziness and headaches, and may also impair the ability to achieve or maintain an erection. It is advisable to limit alcohol intake while taking Cialis.

Always inform your healthcare provider about any medications, supplements, or herbal products you are using to ensure safe and effective treatment with Cialis. If you are prescribed any new medications, check with your provider to avoid potential interactions

Who Should Avoid Cialis?

In this chapter, we will discuss individuals who should avoid using Cialis. While the medication is effective for many, certain health conditions or medications may increase the risk of adverse effects. It's important to be aware of who should refrain from using this treatment.

1. Individuals with Severe Heart Conditions

People with severe heart conditions, such as recent heart attack, stroke, or unstable angina, should avoid Cialis. This includes those with low blood pressure (hypotension) or those who take medications containing nitrates. Cialis may further lower blood pressure, which could lead to dizziness, fainting, or more serious cardiovascular events.

2. Those with Severe Liver or Kidney Disorders

Individuals with severe liver disease or kidney impairment should avoid using Cialis or use it with caution, as the drug is metabolized in the liver and excreted by the kidneys. These conditions may lead to an accumulation of the drug in the bloodstream, increasing the risk of side effects.

3. Those with a History of Priapism

Priapism, a prolonged and painful erection lasting more than four hours, is a rare but serious condition. Individuals with a history of priapism or other blood cell disorders, such as sickle cell anemia, leukemia, or multiple myeloma, should avoid Cialis, as they are at a higher risk of developing this condition.

4. People with Severe Retinal Disorders

Cialis should be avoided by individuals with certain eye conditions, such as retinitis pigmentosa, which is a rare inherited condition that affects the retina. The medication may increase the risk of vision problems in those with such conditions.

5. Those Taking Nitrate Medications

As mentioned earlier, taking Cialis with nitrate medications (e.g., nitroglycerin, isosorbide dinitrate) can lead to a dangerous drop in blood pressure. This combination should be strictly avoided due to the risk of severe hypotension.

6. Those with Allergies to Cialis or its Ingredients

People who are allergic to tadalafil (the active ingredient in Cialis) or any other component of the medication should not take it. Allergic reactions could include rash, swelling, or difficulty breathing, and medical assistance should be sought immediately if these occur.

7. Individuals Under 18 or Over 65

Cialis is not intended for use in individuals under 18. While the medication can be prescribed to men over 65, special considerations are required for dosage adjustments. Older adults may experience more pronounced side effects, and a lower starting dose is often recommended.

8. Those with Deformities of the Penis

If you have a physical deformation of the penis or Peyronie's disease (a condition that causes curved, painful erections), Cialis may not be suitable. Consult with your healthcare provider to explore other treatment options.

Before starting treatment with Cialis, it is essential to discuss your full medical history and any current medications with your healthcare provider to ensure that it is safe for you to use.

Lifestyle Considerations

In this chapter, we will explore the lifestyle factors that can influence the effectiveness and safety of Cialis. While the medication can be a helpful treatment for erectile dysfunction (ED) and benign prostatic hyperplasia (BPH), adopting certain lifestyle changes can support overall health and improve the medication's benefits.

1. **Diet and Nutrition**

A balanced diet plays a crucial role in managing erectile dysfunction. A heart-healthy diet rich in fruits, vegetables, whole grains, lean proteins, and healthy fats can promote better cardiovascular health, which in turn may enhance the effectiveness of Cialis. Foods high in antioxidants, such as berries and leafy greens, can improve blood flow, while excessive consumption of alcohol, caffeine, or highly processed foods may hinder circulation and reduce the effectiveness of medications like Cialis.

2. **Exercise and Physical Activity**

Regular physical activity is another important factor for improving erectile function. Cardiovascular exercises, such as walking, running, and swimming, help improve blood flow and circulation, which is essential for achieving and maintaining an erection. Exercise also helps manage underlying conditions like diabetes and hypertension, which can contribute to ED. A well-rounded fitness routine, including strength training, flexibility exercises, and aerobic activities, can enhance overall health and the success of treatments like Cialis.

3. **Weight Management**

Maintaining a healthy weight can positively impact erectile function. Obesity is often linked to conditions such as diabetes, high blood pressure, and low testosterone, all of which can contribute to erectile dysfunction. Achieving and maintaining a healthy weight through a combination of diet and exercise can help improve blood flow, hormone levels, and overall sexual health. Even modest weight loss can have significant benefits for men experiencing ED.

4. Smoking and Alcohol Consumption

Smoking and excessive alcohol consumption can negatively affect erectile function. Smoking damages blood vessels and restricts blood flow to the penis, while alcohol, when consumed in excess, can impair sexual performance. Reducing or eliminating smoking and limiting alcohol intake can help improve the effectiveness of Cialis and enhance overall sexual well-being.

5. Stress and Mental Health

Stress, anxiety, and depression are significant contributors to erectile dysfunction. Mental health has a direct impact on sexual performance, and chronic stress can lead to or worsen ED. Finding ways to manage stress, such as practicing mindfulness, engaging in relaxation techniques, or seeking therapy, can improve both emotional well-being and sexual health. Counseling or therapy may also be beneficial for those with performance anxiety or relationship-related concerns affecting sexual function.

6. Sleep and Rest

Getting sufficient sleep is vital for overall health and sexual function. Poor sleep quality or sleep disorders, such as sleep apnea, can interfere with hormone levels and lead to fatigue, which in turn may affect erectile function. Aiming for 7-9 hours of quality sleep each night can improve energy levels, mood, and sexual performance, which supports the benefits of Cialis.

7. Managing Chronic Health Conditions

Chronic conditions, such as diabetes, hypertension, and high cholesterol, are closely linked to erectile dysfunction. Managing these conditions through medication, lifestyle changes, and regular check-ups can reduce the impact on sexual health and improve the outcomes of Cialis treatment. Regular visits to healthcare providers for monitoring and adjustments to treatment plans can help prevent complications and improve erectile function.

8. Medication Adherence

Taking Cialis as prescribed and following your healthcare provider's guidance is essential for achieving optimal results. Skipping doses, overuse, or combining Cialis with other medications not recommended by your doctor can lead to ineffective treatment or increase the risk of side effects. Always follow the prescribed dosage and consult your doctor if you have any concerns about your treatment plan.

Incorporating these lifestyle considerations can enhance the effectiveness of Cialis, improve overall health, and contribute to a better quality of life. Always consult a healthcare provider for personalized recommendations tailored to your individual health needs.

Age Considerations When Using Cialis

In this chapter, we explore the age-related factors that may influence the use of Cialis (tadalafil). Understanding these considerations ensures the medication is used safely and effectively across different age groups.

Cialis is typically prescribed for adults aged 18 and above. For younger individuals experiencing erectile dysfunction (ED), it is essential to investigate underlying causes such as psychological stress, lifestyle factors, or medical conditions before initiating treatment. Cialis should only be used under medical supervision after a thorough evaluation.

For men in their 40s and 50s, ED may result from health issues such as diabetes, high blood pressure, or hormonal changes. Cialis can be an effective option, but this age group may also require additional tests, such as cardiovascular assessments, to ensure safety, especially if they have pre-existing conditions.

Men over the age of 65 can use Cialis, but adjustments to the dosage may be necessary. Age-related declines in kidney and liver function can affect how the body processes the medication, increasing the risk of side effects. A lower starting dose is often recommended for older adults to minimize potential risks.

Cialis is not intended for children or teenagers and should only be used by adults with a prescription. Regardless of age, individuals should consult their healthcare provider before starting Cialis, especially if they have chronic medical conditions, take other medications, or experience any unusual symptoms.

How to Track Your Response to Cialis

In this chapter, we will discuss how to effectively track your response to Cialis to ensure that the medication is working as expected and to monitor for any potential side effects. Tracking your response can help you and your healthcare provider make informed decisions about your treatment plan.

1. Keep a Symptom Diary

One of the simplest ways to track your response to Cialis is by maintaining a symptom diary. Record the following information:

- **Effectiveness**: How well Cialis is helping with your erectile dysfunction. Rate your ability to achieve and maintain an erection before and after taking the medication.

- **Side Effects**: Note any side effects you experience, such as headaches, dizziness, or indigestion. Record the severity and duration of these effects.

- **Timing**: Write down when you take Cialis and how long it takes to feel the effects. This can help you assess how well the drug works for you in terms of timing and consistency.

- **Partner Feedback**: If applicable, ask your partner about any noticeable improvements or changes in sexual performance. Feedback from a partner can provide valuable insights.

2. Assessing Overall Well-Being

Your overall well-being can also be an indicator of how well the medication is working. If you feel increased confidence, improved mood, or an enhancement in your relationship due to better sexual function, these are positive signs that the treatment may be effective. On the other hand, if you experience fatigue, anxiety, or other emotional changes, it may be helpful to discuss these with your doctor.

3. Regular Follow-Up Appointments

Regular follow-up appointments with your healthcare provider are important to track the long-term effects of Cialis and make any necessary adjustments. During these visits, your doctor may assess the effectiveness of the medication, monitor side effects, and check for any interactions with other medications you may be taking. These appointments provide an opportunity to adjust your dosage or explore alternative treatments if necessary.

4. Communicate with Your Healthcare Provider

Keep an open line of communication with your healthcare provider throughout your treatment with Cialis. Inform them about any changes in your symptoms, any new side effects you experience, or if the medication does not seem to be working as expected. Your healthcare provider may suggest adjustments in dosage, lifestyle changes, or additional treatments to enhance your results.

Tracking your response to Cialis allows for better management of erectile dysfunction and ensures that the medication is used safely and effectively. Regular monitoring, both independently and with the support of a healthcare provider, is key to achieving the best possible outcomes from treatment.

Tests to Consider

In this chapter, we discuss the essential medical evaluations to consider before starting Cialis (tadalafil). These tests ensure the medication is safe for you and tailored to your health needs, reducing the risk of complications.

1. Cardiovascular Assessment
Since Cialis affects blood flow and can impact blood pressure, it is important to evaluate your heart health. A physical examination, along with tests such as an electrocardiogram (ECG) or stress tests, can help determine if your heart can handle the increased physical activity associated with sexual activity. This is especially important for individuals with a history of heart disease, angina, or hypertension.

2. Blood Pressure Check
Monitoring your blood pressure is critical, as Cialis may

lower blood pressure. Those with pre-existing hypotension or taking medications for hypertension should discuss potential interactions with their doctor.

3. Hormonal Testing
For individuals experiencing erectile dysfunction, hormonal imbalances such as low testosterone levels may be a contributing factor. Blood tests to measure testosterone and other hormone levels can help identify underlying issues that might need treatment alongside Cialis.

4. Kidney and Liver Function Tests
The liver and kidneys play a vital role in metabolizing and excreting Cialis. Blood tests to assess kidney and liver function can help ensure these organs are working effectively, reducing the risk of adverse effects or drug accumulation in the body.

5. Vision and Eye Health Evaluation
While rare, Cialis has been associated with vision changes and conditions like non-arteritic anterior ischemic optic neuropathy (NAION). Individuals with pre-existing eye conditions or a history of vision

problems should undergo a detailed eye examination before using the medication.

6. Comprehensive Medication Review
A review of all current medications and supplements is essential to identify potential drug interactions. This includes nitrates, alpha-blockers, and other medications that may interact with Cialis, causing adverse effects.

Consult with a healthcare professional to ensure that Cialis is a safe and effective option tailored to your health profile. Always follow your doctor's advice and undergo routine health monitoring while using this medication.

Setting Realistic Expectations

In this chapter, we will discuss how to set realistic expectations when using Cialis for erectile dysfunction (ED). While Cialis is an effective treatment for many men, it is important to understand that results can vary, and there are several factors that influence its effectiveness. Setting realistic expectations ensures a more positive and informed experience with the medication.

1. Understanding the Medication's Purpose

Cialis is designed to help men achieve and maintain an erection by increasing blood flow to the penis in response to sexual stimulation. However, it does not directly cause an erection without sexual arousal. It is important to remember that Cialis is not a cure for erectile dysfunction but rather a tool to help manage the symptoms. Expectations should be focused on improving sexual performance rather than expecting a complete reversal of all ED symptoms.

2. Individual Response Varies

Not every individual will experience the same results with Cialis. While some men may see significant improvement in their ability to maintain an erection, others may experience less dramatic changes. Factors such as age, the severity of ED, underlying health conditions, and overall lifestyle choices can influence how well Cialis works. Setting realistic expectations means understanding that while the medication is effective for many, it may not work for everyone in the same way.

3. Onset and Duration of Action

Cialis is known for its long duration of action, lasting up to 36 hours, which gives users flexibility in planning sexual activity. However, the time it takes for the drug to take effect can vary. Some individuals may notice an improvement within 30 minutes to an hour, while others may require more time. The effects of Cialis are not instantaneous, and its timing can be influenced by factors such as food intake or alcohol consumption.

4. Managing Side Effects

Like any medication, Cialis may cause side effects in some individuals. Common side effects include headaches, back pain, or indigestion. These effects are generally mild and subside over time, but they can affect the overall experience of using the medication. Setting realistic expectations involves understanding that side effects may occur and being prepared to address them if they arise.

5. Complementary Lifestyle Changes

While Cialis can enhance sexual performance, it is most effective when used in combination with healthy lifestyle choices. Regular exercise, a balanced diet, and stress management can contribute to better results. Setting realistic expectations means acknowledging that medication alone may not be sufficient if underlying health issues, such as poor cardiovascular health or psychological factors, are not also addressed.

6. Emotional and Psychological Factors

Erectile dysfunction can have a significant emotional and psychological impact. It may cause stress, anxiety, or feelings of inadequacy. Setting realistic expectations with Cialis also involves understanding that while the medication may help with physical symptoms, addressing emotional and psychological factors through counseling or therapy can be an important part of treatment.

7. Open Communication with Healthcare Providers

It is essential to maintain open communication with your healthcare provider about your experiences with Cialis. If the medication is not providing the desired results, a healthcare provider can help adjust the dosage, suggest alternative treatments, or explore other potential causes of ED. Regular check-ins can ensure that expectations are aligned with the reality of the treatment process.

setting realistic expectations when using Cialis involves understanding its intended purpose, recognizing individual variability in response, and considering complementary lifestyle changes and emotional well-being. By taking a balanced approach, individuals can maximize the benefits of Cialis while maintaining a positive and realistic outlook.

Storage and Handling

In this chapter, we will focus on how to properly store and handle Cialis (tadalafil) to maintain its effectiveness and ensure safety. Proper storage is crucial for preserving the quality of the medication, preventing degradation, and ensuring that it works as intended.

1. Storage Temperature

Cialis should be stored at room temperature, typically between 68°F and 77°F (20°C to 25°C). Avoid exposing the medication to extreme temperatures, such as excessive heat or freezing conditions. Storing Cialis outside of these temperature ranges can affect the integrity of the active ingredient and may reduce the medication's effectiveness.

2. Keep in Original Packaging

To protect Cialis from moisture and light, it is best to store it in its original packaging. The blister pack or bottle is designed to shield the medication from environmental factors that could cause it to break down. Always keep the packaging closed and sealed when not in use.

3. Protect from Moisture

Humidity and moisture can affect the quality of Cialis, so it should be stored in a dry place. Avoid storing the medication in bathrooms, where humidity levels can fluctuate significantly. A dry, cool area such as a cupboard or a medicine drawer is ideal.

4. Keep Out of Reach of Children

As with all medications, Cialis should be kept out of the reach of children. Store it in a secure location, preferably in a locked cabinet, to prevent accidental ingestion. Children should never be allowed to access any prescription medications without adult supervision.

5. Avoid Storing in High-Risk Areas

Do not store Cialis in areas exposed to direct sunlight or where it might be subjected to physical damage, such as in a car or near a window. Excessive exposure to sunlight or physical impact could alter the pill's chemical structure.

6. Disposal of Expired or Unused Medication

It is important to properly dispose of any expired or unused Cialis. Do not flush medications down the toilet or pour them into a drain unless instructed to do so by your healthcare provider or pharmacist. Instead, follow proper medication disposal guidelines available at local pharmacies or disposal sites to prevent harm to the environment or unintended exposure.

7. Check for Signs of Degradation

Before taking Cialis, check the pills for any signs of degradation, such as discoloration, cracks, or unusual odors. If any abnormalities are present, discard the medication and consult a healthcare provider for a replacement.

Conclusion

We have explored the essential aspects of erectile dysfunction (ED) and how Cialis (tadalafil) can serve as a treatment option for many individuals. ED is a common condition that can significantly impact a person's quality of life, affecting not only sexual health but also overall well-being and self-esteem. While there are various causes of ED, including physical, psychological, and lifestyle factors, understanding these contributing factors is crucial for choosing the most appropriate treatment.

This guide has aimed to provide a comprehensive overview of Cialis, focusing on its mechanism of action, dosage guidelines, potential side effects, and lifestyle considerations. We also emphasized the importance of consulting with a healthcare provider before beginning treatment with Cialis, as individual health conditions and concurrent medications can impact the suitability and safety of the medication.

It is important to remember that Cialis may not be the right choice for everyone. ED treatment is highly personalized, and a healthcare provider is the best resource to assess the most suitable approach for each individual. A thorough evaluation of your medical history, current health status, and any underlying conditions is essential before starting any medication.

By adhering to the guidelines outlined in this guide and engaging in open communication with a healthcare provider, individuals can make informed decisions about their treatment options and take proactive steps to manage ED effectively. Ultimately, Cialis can be a valuable tool for those who require it, but professional guidance remains crucial for ensuring both safety and effectiveness

It is essential to seek professional advice before starting Cialis or any other medication for ED. Your healthcare provider will help determine the most appropriate treatment based on your specific health needs, lifestyle, and goals.

Made in the USA
Las Vegas, NV
30 November 2024